SKIN RASHES AND HIVES

Effective Strategies for Relief and Prevention.

Joyce O. Kells

Table of Contents

INTRODUCTION

Overview of Skin Rashes and Hives

Skin rashes and hives are common dermatological conditions that can affect people of all ages. People can manage these disorders more effectively and know when to seek medical counsel if they have a thorough understanding of the conditions, symptoms, causes, and treatments. We will discuss what skin rashes and hives are, possible triggers, and identification and treatment methods.

Skin Rashes

Definition: Skin rashes are changes in the texture, color, or appearance of the skin. They may cause itching, burning, or discomfort and manifest as red, inflammatory patches, lumps, or lesions.

Common Types: Eczema (atopic dermatitis), contact dermatitis, psoriasis, heat rash (miliaria), and medication rash are among the common types of skin rashes. Every kind has a unique combination of symptoms and triggers.

Potential Causes: Allergens (plants, animals, foods), irritants (chemicals, detergents), infections (bacterial, viral, fungal), and autoimmune disorders are a few of the variables that might result in skin rashes. Stress and variations in the weather might also be factors.

Symptoms: Depending on the kind and cause, skin rashes can have various symptoms. Redness, itching, swelling, flaking, or peeling skin are typical symptoms. Rashes occasionally come with blisters, pus, or other discharge.

Hives (Urticaria)

Definition: Hives, also known as urticaria, are red, raised, itchy welts on the skin. They can be of any size or shape, and they frequently vanish in a few hours or days after making an abrupt appearance.

Potential Causes: Food allergies, medications, insect stings, and environmental allergens like pollen or pet dander are common causes of hives. Some people may also have hives in response to stress, physical activity, or temperature changes.

Symptoms: The emergence of red, elevated welts that are frequently accompanied by itching is the main sign of hives. These welts can be acute (lasting less than six weeks) or chronic (lasting more than six weeks), and they can move over the body.

Managing Skin Rashes and Hives.

Home Remedies: Cool compresses, soothing ointments, or antihistamines are a few examples of home remedies that can be used to treat a variety of skin rashes and hives. It's also critical to stay away from allergies and recognized triggers.

When to See a Dermatologist: It's crucial to get medical attention if skin rashes or hives develop, persist, or are accompanied by other worrisome symptoms (including breathing difficulties or swelling). A dermatologist can offer a qualified diagnosis and suggest suitable courses of action.

Preventative Measures: Avoiding known triggers and using gentle, fragrance-free skincare products are two recommended skincare practices that can help prevent flare-ups. Overall skin health is also influenced by leading a healthy lifestyle and drinking plenty of water.

Importance of Early Detection and Management

For several reasons, it is vital to identify and treat skin rashes and hives as soon as possible. This is because prompt action can greatly enhance results and lower the risk of consequences. Here's why early detection and management are essential:

- Accurate Diagnosis: Timely detection facilitates a more precise diagnosis, aiding in the determination of the root cause of the rash or hives. This can help direct treatment choices and keep the illness from getting worse.
- Prevention of Complications: Timely medical attention can help avoid consequences like infection, scarring, or exacerbation of symptoms. Early treatment can save lives when severe allergic reactions result in hives.
- Symptom Relief: Itching, redness, and swelling are among the uncomfortable symptoms that can be quickly relieved by treating rashes and hives as soon as possible.
  In addition to enhancing quality of life, this can stop scratching, which can cause skin damage.
- Identification of Triggers: Prompt detection aids in locating possible allergens or triggers that might be the source of the skin problem. By avoiding these triggers, the condition can be properly managed and recurrence can be avoided.
- Prevention of Chronic illnesses: If left untreated, certain skin rashes and hives can turn into chronic illnesses. Prompt management can enhance long-term results and reduce the chance of chronicity.
- Avoiding Misdiagnosis: Appropriate treatment can be ensured, avoidance of needless or potentially dangerous treatments can be avoided, and misdiagnosis or self-diagnosis can be avoided with early detection and professional assessment.

▷ <u>Tracking Development</u>: Prompt management facilitates enhanced tracking of advancement and reaction to therapy. Better results can be achieved by more effectively modifying treatment regimens.

▷ <u>Emotional and Psychological Health</u>: Early treatment of rashes and hives helps reduce tension and anxiety associated with the disease. Improving emotional stability and self-confidence can also be achieved by reducing outward symptoms.

▷ <u>Improved Long-Term Health</u>: Since skin health is intimately related to immune function and other body systems, treating skin disorders early on can help to improve overall health.

When to Seek Medical Help

To ensure appropriate diagnosis and treatment for skin rashes and hives, it's critical to understand when to seek medical attention, particularly if the disease is severe or may be a sign of an underlying medical condition.

CHAPTER 1

UNDERSTANDING SKIN RASHES AND HIVES

This chapter explores the various kinds of skin rashes and hives, as well as their typical symptoms and prevalent causes.

Skin Rashes

Skin rashes are changes in the texture, color, or appearance of the skin. They may cause itching, burning, or discomfort and manifest as red, inflammatory patches, lumps, or lesions.

Types of Skin Rashes

1. Contact Dermatitis

A form of skin rash known as contact dermatitis develops when the skin comes into contact with something that irritates it or triggers an allergic reaction. There are two main types of contact dermatitis; Irritant and Allergic Contact Dermatitis.

> Irritant Contact Dermatitis

A type of skin rash known as "irritant contact dermatitis" develops when an irritating material comes into contact with the skin. Irritating contact dermatitis is a direct reaction to a material that harms the skin, as opposed to allergic contact dermatitis, which is brought on by an immunological response.

Causes

- Exposure to harsh chemicals, such as detergents, solvents, acids, or cleaning agents, is a common cause.
- Extended contact with water, rough surfaces, or particular textiles may cause skin irritation.
- Industrial chemicals, skincare products, and hair dyes are additional possible allergens.

Symptoms

- The impacted region could turn red, dry, and irritated.
- The skin could feel constricted, scorching, or stinging.
- Severe blistering, cracking, or peeling skin are possible outcomes.
- After coming into contact with the irritant, symptoms may arise quickly or they may take longer.

Management.

Identify and Avoid Triggers: The first step in controlling and averting more exposure is determining which irritant is triggering the reaction.

Protective Measures: When working with known irritants, wear gloves, protective clothes, or barrier creams.

Gentle Cleaning: To get rid of the irritation, wash the afflicted region with water and gentle soap.

Soothing Treatments: To calm the skin and lessen inflammation, apply cool compresses or emollients.

<u>Topical Treatments</u>: Hydrocortisone cream available over-the-counter can help reduce irritation and inflammation.

When to Get Medical Assistance:

- If home remedies fail to relieve the rash or if it gets worse.
- If there are indications of infection, such as increasing redness, swelling, or pus in the affected area.
- If the rash spreads widely or starts to interfere with your day-to-day activities.

> Allergic Contact Dermatitis

When an allergen comes into touch with the skin, the immune system reacts, resulting in allergic contact dermatitis. The reaction can vary in severity depending on the sensitivity of the individual and the type of allergen.

Causes:

- Exposure to allergens, such as some metals (like nickel), plants (like poison ivy, poison oak, or poison sumac), rubber, dyes, scents, or preservatives present in cosmetics and personal care items, can cause allergic contact dermatitis.
- Other compounds applied topically or drugs, including antibiotic creams, may also be the reason.

Symptoms:

- The rash typically manifests as red, irritated, and inflamed skin, which may form blisters or pimples that contain clear fluid.
- The impacted region could also get crusty or bloated.
- It may take several hours to many days for symptoms to appear following allergen exposure.
- The location of the allergen's skin contact with the skin usually determines the pattern of the rash.

Management:

<u>Identify and Avoid Allergens</u>: Find out what items trigger your allergic reaction and steer clear of them at all costs.

<u>Wash the Affected Area</u>: As soon as possible after exposure, wash the skin to get rid of any residual allergen by using mild soap and water.

<u>Soothing Treatments</u>: To relieve sensitive skin, apply calamine lotion or cool compresses.

<u>Topical Treatments</u>: Hydrocortisone cream available over-the-counter helps lessen itching and inflammation.

<u>Antihistamines:</u> Oral antihistamines can reduce allergy symptoms such as itching.

When to Get Medical Assistance

- If home remedies are ineffective for the symptoms or if the rash extends to other body areas.
- If there are signs of infection, such as increased redness, warmth, swelling, or pus, or if the rash is severe.
- Should you encounter systemic symptoms, such as dyspnea or facial, lip, or throat swelling, promptly seek emergency medical attention.

2. Atopic Dermatitis (Eczema)

Eczema, also referred to as atopic dermatitis, is a chronic inflammatory skin disorder that results in dry, itchy, and inflammatory skin. It is one of the most prevalent skin disorders in the world and, while it can strike at any age, usually first manifests in childhood.

Causes.

- Genetics: Eczema is associated with a confluence of environmental and genetic variables and frequently runs in families.
- Immune System: Inflammation and flare-ups may result from an overreaction of the immune system to environmental stimuli.
- Skin Barrier Dysfunction: Eczema sufferers may have a weakened skin barrier, which leaves them more vulnerable to allergens and irritants.

- Triggers: Typical triggers include irritants like specific materials or chemicals, dry skin, tension, perspiration, and harsh soaps.

Symptoms.

- Dryness and Itching: The skin gets extremely itchy, scaly, and dry.
- Redness and Inflammation: There may be redness and inflammation in the skin, especially in the face, neck, and flexures (knees and elbows).
- Rashes and Bumps: There may be elevated lumps, blisters, or sores that ooze fluid.
- Cracking and Scaling: Severe cases may cause the skin to crack, which can hurt and increase the chance of infection.

Management.

Moisturizers: Applying emollients and moisturizers regularly helps preserve skin hydrated and fortify the skin barrier.

Topical Treatments: Non-steroidal anti-inflammatory lotions and corticosteroids, whether prescribed or purchased over-the-counter, can help lessen irritation and inflammation.

Bathing Routine: To prevent additional skin irritation, take quick, lukewarm baths and use gentle soaps or cleansers.

Identify and Avoid Triggers: Keep a list of possible triggers, such as particular meals, materials, and irritants, and make an effort to stay away from them.

<u>Antihistamines:</u> Taking an oral antihistamine at night can help reduce itching.

<u>Lifestyle Modifications:</u> Wearing breathable, comfortable clothing and practicing stress management are two other ways to assist control of eczema.

When to Seek Medical Help:

- If symptoms are severe, persistent, or interfering with daily life, seek medical advice for possible prescription treatments.
- If signs of infection (such as increased redness, warmth, or pus) develop, seek medical help promptly.
- In cases of recurring flare-ups or difficulty controlling symptoms, consulting a dermatologist can help develop a personalized treatment plan.

3. Psoriasis

Psoriasis is a chronic inflammatory skin illness that causes skin cells to proliferate and accumulate quickly, resulting in skin that is scaly and irritated in some areas. This condition can vary in severity and may come and go in cycles, with periods of flare-ups followed by periods of remission.

Causes.

- Genetics: Psoriasis appears to have a hereditary component, as the ailment tends to run in families.
- Immune System: Psoriasis is an autoimmune disease, which means that healthy skin cells are wrongly attacked by the immune system, which leads to their rapid multiplication.
- Triggers: Stress, infections, skin injuries, certain drugs, and cold, dry weather are common causes of psoriasis flare-ups.

Types of Psoriasis

- Plaque Psoriasis: The most prevalent kind, distinguished by red, elevated skin areas coated in silvery-white scales. The scalp, knees, elbows, and lower back are common places for these plaques to develop.
- Guttate Psoriasis: Usually follows a streptococcal infection, this condition manifests as tiny, red, drop-shaped lesions. Young adults and children are frequently impacted.
- Pustular Psoriasis: This type of psoriasis, which can affect specific sections of the body (such the hands and feet) or the entire body, is characterized by white pustules surrounded by red skin.
- Inverse Psoriasis: Causes red, shiny, smooth lesions in skin folds like the groin, under the breasts, and the armpits.

- Erythrodermic Psoriasis: An uncommon yet severe type that causes the skin to peel and turn red all over. It needs to be treated right away since it may be fatal.
- Nail Psoriasis: Causes pitting, discoloration, and textural changes in the nails.

Symptoms

- Red Patches: Red, inflamed areas covered with silvery-white scales.
- Itching and Discomfort: The affected skin may itch or be painful, especially when plaques crack or become inflamed.
- Thickened Nails: Changes in the nails, such as thickening, discoloration, or separation from the nail bed.
- Joint Pain: In some cases, joint pain may accompany psoriasis (psoriatic arthritis).

Management

Topical Treatments: To lessen inflammation and scaling, they include coal tar preparations, vitamin D analogs, and corticosteroids.

Phototherapy: Using ultraviolet (UV) light therapy, you can reduce the rate at which skin cells proliferate and alleviate symptoms.

<u>Systemic Treatments</u>: Drugs that inhibit the immune system or control inflammation may be provided orally or intravenously for severe instances.

<u>Lifestyle Modifications</u>: Reducing stress, eating a balanced diet, and staying away from known triggers are all helpful in managing symptoms.

<u>Moisturizers</u>: Applying moisturizers regularly will help lessen scaling and dryness.

When to Get Medical Assistance

- See a doctor for advice on the best course of action if your symptoms worsen, if you have joint pain or other indications of psoriatic arthritis, or if your symptoms worsen.
- Seek medical advice if the ailment is impairing your quality of life or causing you great suffering.

4. Seborrheic Dermatitis

A common skin condition called seborrheic dermatitis results in greasy, red, and scaly spots on the skin. It typically affects the scalp, face, and chest since these regions have a higher density of oil glands. A moderate variation of seborrheic dermatitis that mostly affects the scalp is called dandruff.

Causes

- Overactive Oil Glands: The disorder may be exacerbated by increased sebum (skin oil) production.
- Malassezia Yeast: In certain people, the presence of Malassezia yeast on the skin might result in seborrheic dermatitis.
- Genetics: Seborrheic dermatitis may have a genetic predisposition.
- Other Factors: The severity of seborrheic dermatitis can be influenced by stress, hormonal fluctuations, and specific medical diseases (such HIV or Parkinson's disease).

Symptoms

- Red Patches: The afflicted regions have an inflammatory red appearance.
- Scaly or Greasy Skin: White or yellowish greasy scales may cover certain patches.
- Dandruff: Scalp flaking that ranges in severity from mild to severe.
- Discomfort or Itching: The afflicted regions may burn or itch.

Common Affected Areas

- Scalp: Scaly, irritated areas with dandruff.
- Face: Red, scaly areas on cheeks, around nose, and between eyebrows.

- Back and Chest: These regions may develop red, scaly patches.

Management.

<u>Gentle Cleaning:</u> To prevent irritation, use mild cleansers, soaps, or shampoos made for sensitive skin.

<u>Medicated Shampoos:</u> Shampoos with zinc pyrithione, ketoconazole, or selenium sulfide as components can help reduce scalp problems.

<u>Topical Treatments:</u> In cases that are more severe, topical medications with prescriptions, such as corticosteroids or antifungal lotions, may be required.

<u>Moisturizers:</u> Using moisturizers can lessen flaking and dryness.

<u>Avoiding Triggers:</u> Make an effort to recognize and steer clear of triggers, such as certain goods or stress that could exacerbate symptoms.

When to Seek Medical Assistance

- If symptoms persist or worsen despite home treatments.
- If signs of infection develop, such as increased redness, warmth, or pus.
- If the condition significantly impacts your daily life.

5. Heat Rash (Miliaria)

Heat rash, sometimes referred to as prickly heat or miliaria, is a skin ailment that arises from perspiration getting lodged in clogged sweat ducts, causing skin discomfort and inflammation. In hot, muggy weather or at times when perspiration is profuse, it is typical.

Causes.

- Blocked Sweat Ducts: When perspiration cannot leave through the surface of the skin, it becomes irritated and inflamed.
- Heat and Humid Weather: High humidity levels and temperatures raise the possibility of heat rash.
- Tight or Non-breathable Clothing: Airflow-restricting clothing can exacerbate heat rash and clogged sweat ducts.

Types of Heat Rash

- <u>Miliaria Crystallina:</u> The least severe type, marked by tiny, transparent blisters that usually don't burn or itch. These blisters typically shatter readily.
- <u>Miliaria Rubra:</u> This form manifests as red, itchy pimples or blisters; it is sometimes referred to as prickly heat. It can feel prickly or stinging and happens deeper under the skin.
- <u>Miliaria Profunda:</u> A less frequent but more severe type that causes firm, flesh-colored lumps deeper within the

skin. It may result in less perspiration and a higher chance of heat exhaustion.

Symptoms

- Red, itchy bumps or blisters, often in areas where clothing rubs against the skin.
- Prickly or stinging sensation in the affected areas.
- The rash commonly appears in folds of the skin, such as under the arms, in the groin, or on the neck.

Management

Cool Down: Move to a cooler environment and allow the skin to cool down.

Loose Clothing: Wear loose, breathable clothing to promote airflow and prevent further irritation.

Keep Skin Dry: Avoid excessive sweating and keep the skin dry.

Soothing Treatments: Apply cooling compresses or calamine lotion to soothe the skin.

Avoid Heavy Creams or Ointments: These can further block the sweat ducts and worsen the condition.

When to Seek Medical Assistance:

- If the heat rash lasts for several days or does not get better with home remedies.
- If there is an infection, as seen by pus, swelling, or increasing redness on the rash.
- In case you encounter any signs of heat exhaustion, like nausea or dizziness, you should consult a doctor right away.

6. Fungus Infections

Numerous fungi that like warm, humid conditions can cause fungal infections on the skin. They may impact various body areas, resulting in a variety of skin disorders with unique symptoms. The most common types of fungal skin infections include ringworm, athlete's foot, and tinea versicolor.

Types of Fungal Skin Infections

I.   Ringworm (Tinea Corporis)

Tinea corporis, another name for Ringworm, is a common fungal illness that affects the body's skin. Despite its name, dermatophyte fungus, which like warm, humid conditions, is the true cause of ringworm.

The scalp, face, hands, feet, and groin are not affected by this type of tinea infection; instead, other parts of the body may be affected.

Causes.

- Fungi: Animals, humans, and soil can all harbor dermatophyte fungi, which are the source of ringworm.
- Transmission: It can spread indirectly through contaminated bedding, clothes, or towels, or directly through skin-to-skin contact with an infected person or animal.

Symptoms.

- Circular Rash: A circular or ring-shaped rash with elevated margins and a distinct center is indicative of ringworm. The outer ring could have bumps or scales.
- Itching: The rash may be uncomfortable and is frequently irritating.
- Location: Although the rash can develop anywhere on the body, it typically affects the arms, legs, or trunk.

Managements

Topical Antifungal Medications: The initial line of treatment is usually over-the-counter antifungal creams, gels, or ointments containing substances like terbinafine, miconazole, or clotrimazole. As instructed, apply the medication to the afflicted area.

Oral Antifungal Drugs: A doctor may give oral antifungal drugs for severe or enduring cases.

<u>Keep Skin Clean and Dry</u>: To stop the growth of fungus, practice good hygiene and keep the affected region dry.

<u>Avoid Tight Clothing:</u> To lessen wetness and irritation, dress loosely and breathe well.

Prevention

- Avoid Direct Contact: Steer clear of infected people or animals while coming into contact with their skin.
- Do Not Share Personal Items: Refrain from sharing gowns, towels, or other personal belongings with ringworm sufferers.
- Clean and Disinfect: Ensure that frequently touched surfaces and objects that might come into contact with contaminated skin are routinely cleaned and disinfected.

When to Seek Medical Assistance:

- If, after two weeks, over-the-counter remedies do not alleviate the symptoms.
- If the rash becomes more painful, spreads, or gets worse.
- If there are any symptoms, including increasing redness, swelling, or pus, that indicate a secondary infection.

II. Athlete's Foot (Tinea Pedis)

A common fungal illness that affects the skin of the feet, especially in the spaces between the toes, is called athlete's foot, or tinea pedis.

It is extremely contagious and is brought on by dermatophyte fungi. Athlete's foot is frequently connected to public places where people go barefoot, such as locker rooms and swimming pools.

Causes

- Fungus: Warm, humid conditions are ideal for the growth of dermatophyte fungus, which are the cause of athlete's foot.
- Transmission: Direct touch with contaminated skin or contact with contaminated surfaces—such as floors, towels, or shoes—allows the infection to spread.

Symptoms.

- Itching: The afflicted area, especially in between the toes, may be quite irritating.
- Redness and Scaling: There may be redness, scaling, and cracking of the skin.
- Blisters: Tiny blisters that leak fluid are possible.
- Skin Peeling or Cracking: On the soles of the feet or frequently in the spaces between the toes, the skin may peel or break.

Management.

Topical Antifungal Medications: Athlete's foot can be treated with over-the-counter antifungal creams, gels, or sprays.

Miconazole, terbinafine, and clotrimazole are typical active components.

<u>Oral Antifungals Medications</u>: Oral antifungal drugs may be prescribed by a healthcare provider in cases that are severe or persistent.

<u>Maintain Dry and Clean Feet</u>: Frequent foot washing and thorough drying are important, especially between the toes.

<u>Socks and Footwear</u>: To keep feet dry, put on moisture-wicking socks and breathable shoes. To give your shoes time to break in, try not to wear the same pair every day.

<u>Refrain from Going Barefoot in Public</u>: Wear sandals or flip-flops in shared spaces like showers and locker rooms.

Prevention

- Do Not Share Personal goods: Avoid sharing shoes, towels, socks, or other potentially infected personal goods.
- Keep Feet Dry: To lessen moisture on the feet, apply foot powder or antiperspirant sprays.
- Wear Breathable Footwear: To avoid becoming very wet, use socks and shoes made of breathable fabrics.

When to Seek Medical Help

- If, after two weeks, over-the-counter remedies do not alleviate symptoms.
- Should the illness become more severe, spread, or cause a great deal of discomfort.

- If there are any symptoms, including increasing redness, swelling, or pus, that indicate a secondary infection.

III. Tinea Versicolor

Tinea versicolor, also known as pityriasis versicolor, is a common fungal skin infection caused by an overgrowth of yeast (Malassezia) on the skin. Although this yeast is normally found on the skin, certain circumstances might cause it to multiply and result in tinea versicolor.

Causes

- Yeast Overgrowth: The overgrowth of Malassezia yeast interferes with the skin's natural pigmentation.
- Warm and Humid Weather: Because warm, humid weather promotes yeast growth, the condition is more prevalent in these conditions.
- Excessive perspiration: Tinea versicolor might develop as a result of increased perspiration.
- Oily Skin: People who have oily skin by nature may be more vulnerable.

Indications

- Discolored Patches: Skin patches may have a different color from the surrounding skin. They might be white, pink, tan, or brown.

- Flake and Scaling: There may be some flaking or scaling in the afflicted areas.
- Scratching: The patches may occasionally itch a little.
- Places: The back, shoulders, upper arms, neck, and chest are the most often impacted regions.

Management

<u>Topical Antifungal Treatments</u>: You can help manage the yeast by using over-the-counter antifungal creams, lotions, or shampoos that contain zinc pyrithione, ketoconazole, or selenium sulfide.

<u>Medications for Oral Antifungals</u>: A healthcare professional may recommend oral antifungal drugs in more serious or ongoing situations.

<u>Sun Protection</u>: Steer clear of prolonged sun exposure as this may tan the areas and make them more apparent.

<u>Reduce Perspiration</u>: Try to avoid perspiration as much as possible, especially when the weather is hot and muggy.

Prevention

<u>Good Hygiene</u>: Take frequent showers and make sure your skin is totally dry to avoid leaving too much moisture on it.

<u>Loose Clothes</u>: To lessen heat and moisture on the skin, dress in loose, breathable clothing.

<u>Prevent Oily Skincare Products:</u> Restrict the amount of greasy or oily skincare products you use.

When to Seek Medical Help

- After a few weeks, if over-the-counter remedies do not relieve the symptoms.
- If the infection becomes more uncomfortable or worsens.
- If there are any symptoms, like increasing redness or pus, that indicate a secondary infection.

7. Drug Rash

A drug eruption, sometimes referred to as a drug rash, is an unfavorable cutaneous reaction brought on by taking medicine. Either a minor reaction or a more severe reaction, like drug hypersensitivity syndrome, may include it. Drug rashes are among the most common side effects of medications and can vary greatly in presentation and severity.

Causes

- Medication: Any medication may result in a rash from the drugs. Antibiotics (including penicillin), nonsteroidal anti-inflammatory medications (NSAIDs), and anticonvulsants are frequently implicated.
- Immune Reaction: An immunological reaction to a medication, whether allergic or non-allergic, can result in a drug rash.

- Start Time: Drug rashes might develop right away when taking a medicine, or they can take days or even weeks to manifest.

Symptoms

- Appearance of Rash: Drug rashes can vary in appearance. They can appear as hives, a red, itchy rash, or more serious reactions including skin peeling or blistering.
- Widespread or Localized: The rash could only affect one spot on the body or it could cover the whole thing.
- Other Symptoms: Other symptoms including fever, joint pain, or facial swelling may appear, depending on how severe the reaction is.

Types of Drug Rashes.

Exanthematous (Morbilliform) Rash: Measles-like red patches resembling exanthematous (morbilliform) rashes are the most prevalent type of drug rash. It can spread to different regions after frequently beginning on the trunk.

Urticarial Rash: Also referred to as hives, these itchy welts can vary in size and come and go quickly.

Stevens - Johnson Syndrome/Toxic Epidermal Necrolysis: Severe, possibly fatal responses involving mucous membrane involvement and widespread blistering and peeling of the skin.

Management.

<u>Stop Medications:</u> Stopping the offending medicine is the main treatment for a drug rash. Before stopping any recommended medicine, speak with your doctor.

<u>Antihistamines:</u> You can get relief from itching by using over-the-counter antihistamines.

<u>Topical Interventions:</u> Itching and inflammation can be lessened with the use of topical corticosteroids.

<u>Oral Corticosteroids:</u> Oral corticosteroids may be used to treat more severe reactions.

When to Get Medical Help

- If you think you may have a drug rash, get help from a doctor, especially if you have other symptoms like fever, edema, or trouble breathing.
- If the rash is blistering or peeling, or if it is severe and extensive.
- Seek emergency medical assistance if you suffer a severe response, such as toxic epidermal necrolysis or Stevens-Johnson syndrome.

8. Rosacea

Rosacea is a long-term skin disorder that mostly affects the face. It manifests as bumps and pustules in addition to redness and visible blood vessels.

Although the precise origin of rosacea is unknown, a mix of immune system, environmental, and genetic factors may be involved. Rosacea can range in severity and is more common in people with pale skin.

Causes

- Genetics: The onset of rosacea may be influenced by a hereditary predisposition.
- Immune System: An excessively reactive immune system could be involved.
- Surrounding Triggers: Spicy meals, alcohol, high or low temperatures, sun exposure, stress, and specific skincare products are common triggers.

Symptoms

- Facial Redness: Prolonged redness in the forehead, cheeks, nose, and chin in the center of the face.
- Visible Blood Vessels: Telangiectasias, or tiny, dilated blood vessels, can be seen on the skin.
- Busses and Pustules: The face may develop red, pus-filled bumps that resemble acne.
- Eye Irritation: Dryness, irritation, and redness of the eyes can be symptoms of ocular rosacea.
- Thickened Skin: Rarely, especially in men, the skin of the nose may thicken and swell (rhinophyma).

Management

<u>Topical Treatments:</u> Metronidazole, azelaic acid, or ivermectin-containing prescription lotions or gels can help lessen bumps and inflammation.

<u>Oral Medications:</u> For more severe cases of inflammation or ocular rosacea, a prescription for an oral antibiotic, such as doxycycline, may be issued.

<u>Laser and Light Therapy</u>: These procedures can aid in the reduction of redness and visible blood vessels.

<u>Lifestyle Modifications:</u> Reducing exposure to well-known triggers, such as alcohol, spicy foods, cold weather, and stress, can help control symptoms.

<u>Sun Protection</u>: Using a broad-spectrum sunscreen with a high SPF on a regular basis can help shield the skin and stop flare-ups.

When to Seek Medical Help

- If you think you may have rosacea, get a professional diagnosis and treatment recommendation.
- Should your symptoms get worse or if the first therapies don't work?
- If you frequently irritate your eyes or if you have additional ocular rosacea symptoms.

9. Pityriasis Rose

A common, self-limiting skin ailment known as pityriasis rosea usually manifests as a unique rash with a recognizable pattern. Though the precise etiology is unknown, it is believed to be related to viral infections, specifically human herpesvirus 6 and 7. It mainly affects children and young people.

Causes

- Possible Viral Origin: Pityriasis rosea may be associated with specific viral infections, such as human herpesvirus 6 and 7, however, the precise cause is unknown.
- Seasonal Variation: The ailment is more prevalent in the spring and fall, which may indicate a connection to seasonal virus infections or environmental variables.

Symptoms

- Herald Patch: A big oval patch of pink or salmon-colored skin with a raised, scaly border is commonly the first sign of the illness, called the "herald patch." Usually, it is seen on the back or trunk.
- Secondary Rash: A secondary rash of smaller oval patches emerges on the body in a few days to weeks. These patches are frequently arranged in a Christmas tree pattern along the lines where the back and chest cleave.
- Itching: Some people may not experience any itching at all, but the rash may be mild to moderately itchy.

- Duration: In most situations, the rash goes away on its own in 6 to 8 weeks, but in other circumstances, it may linger longer.

Management

<u>Symptomatic Relief</u>: Pityriasis rosea is a self-limiting condition, hence the main goal of treatment is to reduce symptoms like itching.

<u>Topical Treatments</u>: Calamine lotion or mild topical corticosteroids can be used to reduce itching.

<u>Antihistamines</u>: You can control itching using over-the-counter antihistamines.

<u>Sunshine Exposure</u>: Avoiding sunburn should be the goal of controlled sunshine exposure as it may hasten the cure of the rash.

<u>Moisturizers</u>: Applying light moisturizers devoid of fragrances can aid in skin soothing.

When to Get Medical Help:

- If the rash doesn't get better after a few weeks.
- If there are any worrisome symptoms, such as fever, enlarged lymph nodes, or joint discomfort, along with the rash.
- If the rash itches or causes a lot of discomfort.

10. Lichen Planus

A chronic inflammatory skin disorder that can also affect the scalp, nails, and mucous membranes is called lichen planus. It is distinguished by its irritating, flat-topped, purplish pimples. Although the precise cause of lichen planus is unknown, immune-mediated responses are considered to be involved.

Causes

- <u>Reaction of the Immune System:</u> It is believed that lichen planus is caused by an immune-mediated response that inflames the skin and other tissues.
- <u>Potential Triggers:</u> Allergens, infections, or drugs may occasionally cause lichen planus, though this is not usually the case.

Symptoms

- Skin Lesions: Flat-topped, polygonal, purplish papules with a fine, white, lacy pattern on the surface known as "Wickham's striae"; these lesions may be glossy.

- Itching: There may be extreme itching in the lesions.

- Membranes Mucous: White spots or sores can result from lichen planus, which affects the mucous membranes in the mouth and vaginal area.

- Changes to the Nails: The illness may result in splitting, thinning, or ridging of the nails.

- Scalp Involvement: Hair loss and scarring may result from lichen planus on the scalp.

Management:

<u>Topical Corticosteroids</u>: These are frequently applied topically to soothe skin irritation and inflammation.

<u>Oral Medications:</u> Prescriptions for immune-modulating drugs or oral corticosteroids may be given in more severe situations.

<u>Phototherapy:</u> Using ultraviolet light therapy, skin problems can be lessened.

<u>Antihistamines:</u> You can get relief from itching by using over-the-counter antihistamines.

<u>Oral Care:</u> If the mouth is affected, symptoms can be controlled by practicing proper dental hygiene and avoiding triggers, such as spicy or acidic foods.

When to Seek Medical Help:

- For an accurate diagnosis and treatment plan, see a healthcare provider if you think you may have lichen planus.

- If the symptoms significantly hinder function or create pain or discomfort.

- If you have side effects including intense itching, excruciating mouth sores, or hair loss.

Hives (Urticaria)

Hives also known as Urticaria, is a common skin illness marked by raised lumps or red, itchy welts. It can continue anywhere from a few hours to several weeks or more, and it can happen in reaction to different causes. There are different types of hives based on their triggers and duration:

1. Acute Urticaria

Acute urticaria, sometimes referred to as acute hives, is a skin ailment that appears as raised bumps on the skin or red, itchy welts that last for less than six weeks. Although allergic reactions are a common cause of the illness, other things like infections or stress can also have an impact. Any portion of the body may be affected by acute urticaria, which can be uncomfortable owing to swelling and itching.

Causes

- Allergic Reactions: Allergens can cause an allergic reaction that results in hives. Examples of allergens include some foods (such as nuts, and shellfish), drugs (like antibiotics), insect stings, and latex exposure.

- Infections: Acute urticaria can be brought on by bacterial or viral diseases, including the common cold, the flu, or strep throat.

- Physical Triggers: Acute hives can be brought on by physical stimulation such as exercise, pressure on the skin, or temperature changes, either way.

- Stress: Anxiety or emotional stress can occasionally cause hives.

- Other Causes: Acute urticaria can also be brought on by some medications, medical disorders, and blood transfusions.

Symptoms

- Red, Itchy Welts: Raised, red welts appear on the skin and may be itchy or cause a burning or stinging sensation.

- Swelling: Angioedema, or swelling, might happen occasionally. It usually affects the hands, feet, lips, and eyes.

- Transient Lesions: Although new welts may emerge in different locations, the welts may appear abruptly and often go away in a few hours.

Managements

<u>Antihistamines:</u> Over-the-counter antihistamines can help reduce swelling and itching. Examples include diphenhydramine, loratadine, and cetirizine.

<u>Avoiding Triggers:</u> Recognizing and staying away from recognized triggers (such as particular foods or drugs) can help avert further episodes.

<u>Topical Treatments:</u> Topical creams or lotions may help relieve localized irritation.

<u>Oral Corticosteroids:</u> Short courses of oral corticosteroids may be recommended to treat symptoms in more severe cases.

When to Seek Medical Assistance.

- If, after a few days, over-the-counter remedies do not relieve hives.

- If you exhibit symptoms indicative of a severe allergic reaction, such as fast heartbeat, facial or throat swelling, or trouble breathing (anaphylaxis). Seek quick emergency medical assistance.

- If you often get hives or exhibit angioedema symptoms.

2. Chronic Urticaria

The skin ailment known as chronic urticaria, or chronic hives, is characterized by raised bumps or red, itchy welts that persist for longer than six weeks. Since the reasons for chronic urticaria are frequently idiopathic (unknown), although in certain situations the condition may be exacerbated by specific triggers, managing the condition can be difficult. The welts might vary in size and shape and can arise anywhere on the body.

Causes

- Idiopathic: Chronic urticaria is also referred to as chronic spontaneous urticaria because the precise etiology is frequently unknown.

- Autoimmune Conditions: In certain instances, autoimmune disorders—disorders in which the body's immune system unintentionally targets its tissues—may be connected to chronic urticaria.

- Physical Triggers: Certain cases could be linked to physical triggers like pressure, heat or cold, sunlight, or physical activity.

- Other Factors: In some cases, foods, drugs, hormonal fluctuations, and persistent infections can all lead to chronic urticaria.

Symptoms

- Red, Itchy Welts: The skin may develop raised, red welts that are extremely uncomfortable. Over time, the welts may appear and disappear, changing in size and shape.

- Swelling: Angioedema, or swelling, might happen occasionally. It usually affects the hands, feet, lips, and eyes.

- Duration: There may be remission and relapse intervals, and symptoms may last for several months or even years.

Management

<u>Antihistamines</u>: The first line of treatment for chronic urticaria is frequently non-drowsy over-the-counter antihistamines like cetirizine or loratadine. In certain situations, higher dosages or prescription antihistamines might be required.

<u>Leukotriene Receptor Antagonists</u>: Some patients may benefit from the usage of medications like montelukast as an adjunctive treatment.

<u>Oral Corticosteroids:</u> To treat severe symptoms, doctors may prescribe brief courses of oral corticosteroids.

<u>Omalizumab</u>: An injectable monoclonal antibody, omalizumab is administered to lessen the frequency and intensity of symptoms in cases that do not respond to previous treatments.

<u>Avoiding Triggers:</u> Flare-ups can be avoided by recognizing and avoiding known triggers.

When to Get Medical Assistance:

- If using over-the-counter remedies or prescription drugs does not relieve symptoms.

- Seek emergency medical assistance right once if hives are accompanied by angioedema or symptoms of a severe allergic response (anaphylaxis).

- If symptoms increase, linger, or have a major negative influence on your quality of life.

3. Physical Urticaria

Physical urticaria is a type of hives (urticaria) triggered by physical stimuli such as pressure, temperature changes, or other external factors. This is a prevalent type of urticaria, with various subtypes existing based on the particular physical cause. Physical urticaria can present with a variety of symptoms, but red, elevated welts and skin itching are frequently seen. Below are the main types of physical urticaria and their characteristics:

I. Dermatographism (Dermatographia)
  - Description: Also referred to as "skin writing," dermatographism is a condition in which pressure or scratching of the skin results in welts and redness.
  - Symptoms: Within minutes of applying pressure, the skin develops linear red markings or hives, which can linger for several minutes to hours.

II. Cold Urticaria
  - Description: Exposure to cold temperatures, whether from cold air, cold water, or cold objects, can cause cold urticaria.

- <u>Symptoms</u>: After being exposed to cold, red, itchy hives frequently develop on the skin within minutes. Usually, symptoms go away when the skin warms up.

III. Heat Urticaria

- Description: Exposure to warm or hot temperatures, such as those found in warm weather, warm water, or sauna heat, can cause heat urticaria.
- Symptoms: Shortly after being exposed to heat, usually within minutes, red, itchy hives develop on the skin. The symptoms can go away when the skin cools.

IV. Cholinergic Urticaria

- Description: Elevation of body temperature, as from physical activity, hot showers, or emotional stress, is the cause of cholinergic urticaria.
- Symptoms: Tiny, red, itchy pimples that frequently have a burning or tingling feeling on the skin surface. Usually, the symptoms go away in an hour.

V. Solar Urticaria

- Description: Sunlight or other UV light sources can cause solar urticaria.
- Symptoms: Within minutes of sun exposure, the skin develops red, itchy hives; these symptoms go away as soon as the exposure ends.

VI. Vibratory Urticaria

- Description: Vibrations, such as those from power tool use or vehicle rides, can cause vibratory urticaria.
- Symptoms: Within minutes of exposure to the vibrations, red, itchy hives develop on the skin.

VII. Delayed Pressure Urticaria

- Description: Prolonged pressure on the skin, such as that which results from carrying heavy objects or wearing tight clothing, is the cause of delayed pressure urticaria.
- Symptoms: A few hours after the exposure, swelling, and soreness appear in the area where the pressure was applied.

Management

<u>Avoid Triggers</u>: Physical urticaria episodes can be avoided by recognizing and avoiding the precise physical triggers.

<u>Antihistamines:</u> Prescription or over-the-counter antihistamines can be used to treat hives and itching.

<u>Prescription Medications:</u> Prescription drugs like omalizumab or leukotriene receptor antagonists may be utilized in extreme situations.

<u>Lifestyle Changes:</u> Keeping the body temperature stable, avoiding tight accessories, and dressing loosely can all help control symptoms.

4. Contact Urticaria

When a chemical that causes an allergic or irritating reaction comes into direct touch with the skin, it can cause contact urticaria, a type of hives. Red, itchy welts or raised bumps on the skin may result from the reaction, and they frequently emerge minutes after coming into contact with the trigger. The duration of contact urticaria might range from a few hours to many days, with varying degrees of severity.

Types of Contact Urticaria

I.   Urticaria with IgE-Mediated Contact

When skin comes into direct contact with an allergen, immunoglobulin E (IgE) antibodies cause an allergic reaction on the skin that results in IgE-mediated contact urticaria, a kind of hives. This type of urticaria is characterized by a rapid onset of symptoms at the site of contact with the allergen.

Causes

- Allergens: Typical allergens that may result in contact urticaria mediated by IgE include:

- Latex: Sensitive people may experience allergic responses to latex gloves and other goods.
- Specific Foods: Certain foods, such as nuts, shellfish, and eggs, can react when they come into direct contact with the skin.
- Animal Dander: Some people may experience responses if they come into contact with animal fur or dander.
- Medication: Some topically applied drugs may result in contact urticaria.

Symptoms

- Rapid Onset: After coming into touch with the allergen, symptoms typically start to show.
- Localized Reaction: The skin at the location of allergen exposure develops red, itchy welts or raised bumps.
- Swelling (Angioedema): The afflicted area, especially the hands, lips, or face, may experience swelling.
- Systemic Symptoms: Severe cases may result in systemic symptoms including breathing problems, lightheadedness, or anaphylaxis.

Management

Avoiding Triggers: IgE-mediated contact urticaria episodes can be avoided by recognizing and avoiding known allergens that trigger reactions.

Antihistamines: Over-the-counter antihistamines can lessen hives and ease itching.

<u>Topical Treatments:</u> Localized discomfort and inflammation can be controlled with mild topical corticosteroids.

<u>Epinephrine Auto-Injector:</u> People who have experienced severe allergic responses in the past may need to keep an epinephrine auto-injector on hand for use in an emergency (such as an EpiPen).

When to Seek Medical Assistance:

- Seek emergency medical assistance right away if you suspect a serious allergic reaction (anaphylaxis), exhibiting symptoms such as breathing difficulties, throat swelling, or loss of consciousness.

- If over-the-counter medications do not relieve the symptoms if they worsen, or if they persist.

- If you get hives or angioedema in several different body parts.

II. Non-IgE-Mediated Contact Urticaria

Non-IgE-mediated contact urticaria is a form of urticaria (hives) that develops when an allergen or irritant comes into touch with the skin and causes a reaction that is not mediated by immunoglobulin E (IgE) antibodies. Alternatively, the reaction could be caused by irritation of the skin directly or by other immune system routes. Compared to IgE-mediated contact urticaria, the start of symptoms is usually delayed, and they may persist longer.

Causes

- Irritants: Non-IgE-mediated contact urticaria can result from direct contact with irritating materials such as solvents, detergents, acids, or alkalis.
- Allergens: Certain allergens, such as certain metals (like nickel), colors, or chemicals in personal care items, can cause a reaction when they come into contact with them.
- Plants: Some plants can induce non-IgE-mediated contact urticaria, including poison ivy, poison oak, and poison sumac.

Symptoms

- Delayed Onset: After coming into contact with the allergen or irritant, symptoms may not appear for hours.
- Localized Reaction: The skin at the point of contact develops red, itchy, and possibly painful welts or raised lumps.
- Swelling: In severe situations, swelling (angioedema) may develop in the affected area.
- Duration: Depending on the chemical involved and the intensity of the reaction, symptoms may last for hours or even days.

Management

<u>Avoiding Triggers:</u> Non-IgE-mediated contact urticaria episodes can be avoided by recognizing and avoiding known allergies or irritants.

<u>Topical Treatments:</u> Topical corticosteroids applied sparingly can help lessen irritation and inflammation.

<u>Antihistamines:</u> You can treat itching and discomfort using over-the-counter antihistamines.

<u>Barrier Protection:</u> When handling allergies or irritants, wearing gloves or protective clothes can help avoid direct skin contact.

When to Seek Medical Assistance

- If using over-the-counter medications does not relieve the symptoms.

- Should symptoms intensify or result in severe discomfort?

- If the affected area shows any indications of infection, such as increasing warmth, redness, or pus.

General Common Causes and Triggers of Rashes and Hives.

Hives and rashes can be brought on by a wide range of variables and can happen for a variety of reasons. Effective management of certain skin disorders can be facilitated by knowledge of common causes and triggers. The general common causes and triggers of rashes and hives are listed below:

1. Allergens

- ▷ Food: Some people may get rashes or hives in response to certain foods, including dairy, eggs, nuts, and seafood.
- ▷ Medications: Certain medications, such as nonsteroidal anti-inflammatory medicines (NSAIDs) and antibiotics (like penicillin), can trigger allergic responses that result in rashes or hives.
- ▷ Environmental Allergens: Mold spores, dust mites, pet dander, and pollen all cause allergic skin reactions.
- ▷ Contact Allergens: Chemicals in personal care items, latex, and some metals (like nickel) can all result in contact dermatitis and hives.

2. Infection

- ▷ Viral Infections: Rashes can occasionally result from common viral diseases like the flu or the common cold.
- ▷ Bacterial Infections: Rashes can result from bacterial illnesses, including skin infections and strep throat.
- ▷ Fungal Infections: Rashes and itching can be brought on by illnesses like athlete's foot or ringworm.

3. Skin Conditions

- ▷ Eczema: Dry, itchy, and inflammatory skin are the hallmarks of this chronic skin disorder.
- ▷ Psoriasis: Red, scaly patches on the skin are a chronic skin ailment.

> Rosacea: A skin ailment that frequently affects the face results in redness and visible blood vessels.

4. Physical Setbacks

> Heat: Certain persons may have rashes or hives in warm weather or after taking a hot bath or shower.
> Cold: In sensitive individuals, exposure to cold air or water might result in cold-induced urticaria.
> Pressure: Tight apparel or accessories may cause pressure or contact urticaria.
> Sunlight: Some persons may develop solar urticaria as a result of sun exposure.

5. Emotions and Stress

> Stress: Skin diseases like eczema or hives can be aggravated or brought on by emotional stress and anxiety.
> Exercise: Certain people may develop cholinergic urticaria as a result of intense physical effort.

6. Autoimmune and Immune System Disorders

> Autoimmune Conditions: Rashes or persistent hives may be a symptom of some autoimmune diseases.
> Immune System Imbalance: Chronic skin disorders may be exacerbated by immune system imbalances.

7. Hormonal Changes

- ▷ Hormonal Fluctuations: Skin abnormalities and rashes can be brought on by fluctuations in hormone levels, such as those that occur during pregnancy, menopause, or menstrual cycles.

Management

- One way to manage rashes and hives is to recognize and stay away from recognized triggers.

- Topical medications and over-the-counter antihistamines can offer relief.

- Seeking advice from a medical professional can assist in identifying the root cause and creating a suitable treatment strategy.

CHAPTER 2

IDENTIFYING YOUR RASH OR HIVES

Identifying the type of rash or hives you are experiencing can help you determine the best course of treatment and whether you should seek medical advice.

Signs and Symptoms

When you have a rash or hives, paying attention to the particular symptoms and indicators can help you diagnose the problem, assess its severity, and choose the best course of action. Here are some crucial indicators and symptoms to be aware of:

1. Redness

- Rash: Examine the skin for any red areas or patches.
- Hives: Raised, red welts or bumps, sometimes surrounded by a pale halo.

2. Itching

- Severity: Itching can be minor to severe and is frequently brought on by rashes and hives.
- Timing: Either constant or sporadic itching is possible, and it may get worse at night.

3. Swelling (Angioedema)

- Localized Swelling: Edema may develop near the site of the injury, especially in the hands, feet, lips, and eyes.
- Severity: The degree of swelling might vary, and it may be accompanied by soreness or pain.

4. Blisters

- Presence of Blisters: Certain rashes may appear as painful or itchy blisters packed with fluid.
- Size and Distribution: Examine the blisters' size and dispersion.

5. Texture

- Rash: Look for textures like lumpy, scaly, or rough skin.
- Hives: The texture of hives is usually smooth.

6. Distribution

- Localized: Ascertain whether the hives or rash are restricted to a single location, such as the arms, legs, face, or neck.
- Widespread: Examine whether the rash or hives are scattered around the body or whether they cover a wide area.

7. Other Symptoms

- Pain: Rashes can sometimes be painful, particularly if they're accompanied by blisters or ulcers.
- Stinging or Burning: Some rashes or hives may have a stinging or burning feeling.
- Additional Systemic Signs: Look for concomitant symptoms including a fever, exhaustion, sore throat, or breathing problems.

8. Changes Over Time

- Duration: Indicate the length of time the rash or hives have persisted.
- Advancement: Keep an eye on whether the rash or hives are becoming worse, changing, or going away on their own.

When to Seek Medical Help

- Seek emergency care right away if breathing becomes difficult or if swelling occurs in the face, tongue, or throat as a result of the rash or hives.

- Should the rash or hives continue, get worse, or cause a lot of discomfort, consult a doctor for a more thorough assessment.

- Seek medical assistance if there are infection-related symptoms, such as fever, pus, increasing redness, or warmth.

Common Appearance of Rashes and Hives

Depending on the underlying cause, rashes and hives can occur in a variety of ways. Identifying the type of rash or hives you may be experiencing might be aided by observing the common symptoms of different skin ailments. Observe the following general characteristics:

Rashes

1. Redness

   - Rashes frequently manifest as pink or red areas on the skin.

   - Depending on the reason, redness might have varying intensities.

2. Texture:

   - Smooth: Certain rashes have smooth, flat patches of skin on them.

   - Rough: People with psoriasis or eczema may have a rough or bumpy texture.

   - Scaly: Some rashes, such as those brought on by psoriasis, might appear scaly.

3. Distribution

- Rashes can be dispersed across the body or restricted to a single spot.

- Some rashes, including those brought on by illnesses, could have a pattern.

4. Blisters

- Fluid-filled blisters, which are common in illnesses like shingles or chickenpox, might accompany some rashes.

5. Crusting

- As blisters break open and dry up, rashes containing blisters may develop crusts.

6. Additional Symptoms

- Itching: Itching can be present with many rashes and can range in intensity.

- Pain: Certain rashes can hurt, particularly if they are accompanied by blisters or ulcers.

Hives (Urticaria)

1. Welts

- Red, elevated welts or bumps on the skin are indicative of hives.

- The welts can occur in groups and range in size and shape.

2. Pale Center

- Hives are distinguished by their unique pale center encircled by a crimson border.

3. Itching

- Hives frequently cause excruciating itching, along with a stinging or burning feeling.

4. Transient

- Although additional welts may emerge in other places, hives usually go away on their own in a few hours. Hives may also appear suddenly.

5. Swelling (Angioedema)

- Hives occasionally coexist with swelling (angioedema) of the lips, tongue, face, or other parts of the body.

When to Seek Medical Help

- Seek emergency care right away if you suffer from excruciating itching, trouble breathing, facial or throat swelling, or any other symptoms of a severe allergic reaction.

- See a healthcare professional for additional assessment and treatment if the rash or hives develop, last longer, or cause you a lot of discomfort.

Self-Evaluation and Monitoring

You can gain a better understanding of your rash or hives, find possible causes, and improve the way you manage your symptoms by self-assessing and tracking. You may give your doctor comprehensive information to help with diagnosis and treatment by keeping track of your health. The following are some actions for tracking and self-evaluation:

1. Keep a Symptom Diary

> Time and Date: Note the onset and end times of your rash or hives.
> Location: Make a note of the particular body parts where the rash or hives develop.
> Appearance: Describe the color, size, form, and texture of the rash or hives as well as how they appear.
> Severity: On a scale of 1 to 10, indicate how severe your symptoms (such as pain, swelling, or itching) are.

> Other Symptoms: Make a note of any additional symptoms you encounter, such as temperature, exhaustion, or breathing problems.

2. Identify Triggers

> Recent Activities: Take into account your activities, such as working out, taking a shower, or being outside, when the rash or hives first started.

> Allergen or Irritant Exposure: Note any possible triggers, such as the use of new skincare products, dietary modifications, or contact with allergens or irritants that are known to cause problems.

> Environmental Factors: Take note of any modifications to the weather, temperature, or humidity in your surroundings.

3. Monitor Duration and Progression

> Duration: Note the length of time the rash or hives persist and the speed at which they go away.

> Progression: Track the spread, appearance change, or localization of the rash or hives.

4. Monitor Treatments and Results

> Medicines: List any prescription or over-the-counter drugs you take, such as topical medicines or antihistamines.

- Home Remedies: Note any remedies you employ at home, along with their outcomes.
- Results: Keep note of any improvements or adverse effects that occur as well as how your symptoms change in response to treatment.

5. Review Personal and Family Medical History

- Pre-existing Conditions: List any allergies or skin conditions you currently have.
- Family History: Take into account if allergies or skin disorders run in the family.

6. Report Your Results to Your Doctor

- Consultation: Give your doctor comprehensive details about your condition by using your symptom diary.
- Medication and Therapy: With the use of this data, your healthcare professional can diagnose you and suggest a customized course of therapy.

CHAPTER 3

HOME REMEDIES FOR SKIN RASHES

Mild skin rashes can frequently be relieved at home with home treatments. It's crucial to remember that these treatments should not be used in place of medical guidance if your rash is severe or persistent and that you should use them carefully if you have sensitive skin or allergies.

Soothing and Moisturizing Treatments

In addition to relieving itching and pain, soothing and moisturizing therapies can assist in keeping skin hydrated and promote healing in cases of skin rashes. Here are some common soothing and moisturizing treatments you can try at home for skin rashes:

1. Gel Aloe Vera

   - How to use it: Two to three times a day, apply pure aloe vera gel straight to the affected region.
   - Benefits: Aloe vera has cooling and anti-inflammatory qualities that assist relieve inflammation and itching.

2. Cocoa Butter

   - How to use it: Apply a tiny bit of virgin coconut oil to the rash and massage it in gently.

- Benefits: Because of its high fatty acid content, hydrating qualities, and anti-inflammatory qualities, coconut oil is good for dry, irritated skin.

3. Shea Butter

- How to Apply: To soothe and hydrate the afflicted region, apply a thin coating of shea butter.
- Benefits: Shea butter is an all-natural moisturizer that has anti-inflammatory and anti-drying properties.

4. Colloidal Oatmeal.

- Usage Instructions: For 15-20 minutes, add finely ground oats, or colloidal oatmeal, to a lukewarm bath and soak.
- Benefits: Because of its calming qualities, oatmeal can help reduce inflammation and itching.

5. Honey

- How to Use: Rinse off the area after a few minutes by applying a thin layer of raw, organic honey.
- Benefits: Honey can relieve inflamed skin because of its antibacterial and anti-inflammatory qualities.

6. Chamomile

- How to Apply: Make chamomile tea, let it cool, then use a cotton ball or towel to apply it to the rash.

- Benefits: The anti-inflammatory and soothing properties of chamomile help reduce inflammation and itching.

7. Calendula Cream

- How to Use It: Administer calendula cream or ointment to the area that is impacted as required.
- Benefits: Calendula has soothing and healing properties that can help calm irritated skin.

8. Avocado Oil

- How to Use It: Apply a tiny bit of avocado oil to the area that is afflicted.
- Benefits: Rich in vitamins and good fats, avocado oil may moisturize and nourish skin.

9. Hydration

- How to Use: Drink lots of water throughout the day to keep the skin well moisturized.
- Benefits: Retaining hydration promotes healing and helps keep skin hydrated.

When to Get Medical Help

- Get help if the rash doesn't go away, gets worse, or exhibits symptoms of infection.

▷ Get emergency medical assistance right once if you suffer breathing difficulties or other symptoms of a severe allergic reaction (anaphylaxis).

Cooling Baths and Compressors

Cooling compresses and baths are effective at relieving itching, irritation, and discomfort, making them useful home treatments for skin rashes. Through the reduction of inflammation and calming of the affected area, these treatments aid in skin soothing. You might try the following common at-home cooling compresses and baths for skin rashes:

1. Cool Compressors

   - How to Apply: Soak a washcloth or clean, soft fabric in cold water. After wringing off extra water, dab the rash with a cool, moist cloth. After 10 to 15 minutes, remove it and repeat as necessary.
   - Benefits: By narrowing blood vessels and calming the skin, cool compresses can help lessen burning, itching, and swelling.

2. Cold Packs:

   - How to Use it: Gently apply a cold pack or ice pack to the affected area for ten to fifteen minutes after wrapping it in a thin cloth.

- Benefits: To ease discomfort and itching, cold packs can help numb the region and reduce inflammation.

3. Colloidal Oatmeal Baths

- How to Use it: To warm bathwater, add colloidal oatmeal, which is made of finely ground oats. Take a 15 to 20-minute bath soak. To prevent further irritation, gently pat the skin dry with a gentle towel.
- Benefits: Because of its anti-inflammatory qualities, colloidal oatmeal can help reduce irritation and itching.

4. Baking Soda Baths

- How to Use: Soak for 15 to 20 minutes in a lukewarm bath after adding 1/4 cup of baking soda.
- Benefits: Baking soda can calm inflamed skin and reduce irritation.

5. Apple Cider Vinegar Baths

- How to Apply: To lukewarm bathwater, add 1/2 to 1 cup of apple cider vinegar. After soaking for fifteen to twenty minutes, rinse with fresh water and pat dry.
- Benefits: Because of its antibacterial and anti-inflammatory qualities, apple cider vinegar may help lessen irritation and itching.

6. Compressed Peppermint Tea

- How to Apply: Make a pot of peppermint tea, let it cool, and then use the liquid to soak a cloth. For a calming effect, apply the cool cloth to the affected area.
- Benefits: Tea with peppermint leaves has a cooling effect on the skin that helps reduce inflammation and itching.

When to Seek Medical Help

- Get help if your rash doesn't go away, gets worse, or exhibits symptoms of an infection, such as increasing warmth, redness, or pus.

- Seek emergency medical attention right away if you suffer from severe allergic reactions (anaphylaxis), such as breathing difficulties.

Natural and Herbal Treatments

It is possible to relieve the symptoms of skin rashes, including redness, irritation, and itching, by using herbal and natural therapies. Use caution when using these cures, especially if you have sensitive skin or allergies, even though they might provide relief. Should you have any questions about utilizing these treatments, always get advice from your healthcare professional. The following are some popular natural and herbal treatments for skin rashes that you can apply at home:

1. Chamomile

- How to Use: Make a cup of chamomile tea, let it cool, then use a cotton ball or towel to apply it to the rash. An alternative is to dilute the essential oil of chamomile in a carrier oil.
- Benefits: Because of its calming and anti-inflammatory qualities, chamomile can help reduce discomfort and itching.

2. Calendula

- How to Apply: On the rash, apply calendula cream or ointment directly. Calendula tea can also be brewed and used as a compress.
- Benefits: Calendula has anti-inflammatory and therapeutic qualities that help soothe inflamed skin.

3. Lavender

- How to Use: Apply lavender essential oil sparingly to the afflicted region after diluting it with carrier oil (like coconut oil).
- Benefits: Lavender can help lessen irritation and itching because of its soothing and anti-inflammatory qualities.

4. Tea Tree Oil

- How to Use: Apply diluted tea tree oil to the rash by diluting it with a carrier oil (such as jojoba or almond oil).

- Benefits: Tea tree oil can help lessen irritation and prevent infection because of its antibacterial and anti-inflammatory qualities.

5. Witch Hazel

- How to Use It: Use a cotton ball or pad to apply witch hazel extract to the rash.
- Benefits: With its astringent and anti-inflammatory qualities, witch hazel can help calm and desiccate the rash.

6. Neem Oil

- How to Apply: Apply neem oil to the afflicted area after diluting it with carrier oil (like olive oil).
- Benefits: Neem oil can relieve and cure rashes because of its antibacterial and anti-inflammatory qualities.

7. Aloe Vera

- How to Use It: Directly apply pure aloe vera gel to the area that is afflicted.
- Benefits: Aloe vera is well-known for its anti-inflammatory, calming, and relaxing qualities.

8. Turmeric Paste

- How to Use: Make a paste out of turmeric powder and water, then apply it on the rash. After a few minutes, leave it on and rinse it off.
- Benefits: Due to its antibacterial and anti-inflammatory qualities, turmeric may aid in the rash's healing.

When to Seek Medical Help

- Get help if your rash doesn't go away, gets worse, or exhibits symptoms of an infection (such as increasing redness, warmth, or pus).

- Seek emergency medical attention right away if you suffer from severe allergic reactions (anaphylaxis), such as breathing difficulties.

Over-The-Counter Treatments (OTC)

Over-the-counter (OTC) medications can be used as efficient home remedies for rashes on the skin, reducing irritation, redness, and itching. These commonly accessible therapies can aid in the management of mild to moderate cutaneous rashes. The following are some popular over-the-counter remedies for rashes on the skin:

1. Hydrocortisone Cream

   - How to Apply: Up to three times a day, apply a thin coating of 1% hydrocortisone cream to the afflicted area.
   - Benefits: A moderate corticosteroid that can help lessen redness, swelling, and itching is hydrocortisone.

2. Calamine Lotion

   - How to Use It: Load the rash with calamine lotion as needed, and let it dry on the skin.
   - Benefits: Calamine lotion relieves inflammation and itching while having a cooling effect.

3. Antihistamines Tablets

   - How to Apply: Follow the advice on the packaging when taking oral antihistamines like cetirizine (Zyrtec), loratadine (Claritin), or diphenhydramine (Benadryl).
   - Benefits: Antihistamines can help with hives or allergic skin rashes by reducing itching and allergic responses.

4. Oatmeal Bath Products

   - How to Use: Soak in a lukewarm bath for 15 to 20 minutes using colloidal oatmeal bath products.
   - Benefits: Products for bathing that contain oatmeal help hydrate and calm the skin, lessening irritation and itching.

5. Moisturizers

- How to Use: Regularly massage the afflicted region with hypoallergenic and fragrance-free moisturizers.
- Benefits: Moisturizers can help shield the skin from dryness and irritation while also keeping it hydrated.

6. Topical Antihistamines

- How to Apply: When necessary, treat the rash with a topical antihistamine cream, such as diphenhydramine.
- Benefits: Localized relief from itching and irritation can be obtained using topical antihistamines.

7. Topical Antifungal Creams

- How to Apply: Use an over-the-counter antifungal cream, such as clotrimazole or miconazole, following the advice on the packaging if a fungal infection is the source of the rash.
- Benefits: These treatments can help treat fungal infections and lessen their accompanying symptoms, like redness and itching.

When to Seek Medical Help

- Seek medical help if the rash worsens or exhibits signs of infection (such as increased redness, warmth, or pus), or if it does not improve with over-the-counter medicines.

- Seek emergency medical attention right away if you suffer from severe allergic reactions (anaphylaxis), such as breathing difficulties.

CHAPTER 4

HOME REMEDIES FOR HIVES

Home remedies can lessen itching, swelling, and discomfort in mild to moderate instances of urticaria, or hives. However, you should get medical attention right away if you have severe hives or any other symptoms of anaphylaxis, such as breathing difficulties or swelling in your face or throat.

Avoiding Known Triggers

An important part of treating hives (urticaria) and averting flare-ups is avoiding recognized triggers. The frequency and intensity of hives can be decreased by recognizing and avoiding certain triggers. Underneath home treatments for hives, the following advice can help you avoid identified triggers:

1. Keep a Symptom Diary

   - Things Note Down: Jot down pertinent information about your location, activities, food, and other experiences related to your hives episodes.
   - Benefits: Over time, this might assist you in recognizing trends and possible triggers.

2. Avoid Food Triggers

- Instructions: Shellfish, nuts, eggs, dairy, and several fruits and vegetables are common food triggers. Keep a diet journal to see which foods tend to trigger hives most frequently.
- Benefits: A recognized dietary trigger's avoidance can help avoid flare-ups of hives.

3. Watch for Medication Triggers

- Instructions: Hives can be brought on by some medications, including antibiotics and nonsteroidal anti-inflammatory drugs (NSAIDs). Make a note of all the drugs you take and how they affect your symptoms.
- Benefits: Keeping away from drugs that cause hives can aid in the management of the illness.

4. Reduce Stress

- Instructions: Engage in stress-relieving activities like yoga, deep breathing exercises, meditation, or consistent exercise.
- Benefits: Handling stress can help stop outbreaks of hives because stress can cause or exacerbate hives.

5. Avoid Environmental Triggers

- Instruction: Pollen, pet dander, dust mites, mold, and insect stings are examples of common environmental triggers. Maintain a clean and allergen-free house.
- Benefits: Reducing exposure to triggers in the environment can help avoid hives.

6. Dress Appropriately

- Instruction: To minimize irritation and stop heat-induced hives, wear loose-fitting, breathable clothing.
- Importance: Wearing clothes that are too tight or too hot can cause hives, so preparing properly can help prevent flare-ups.

7. Be Mindful of Exercise

- Instruction: Certain people may have hives after exercising. If you exercise and have hives afterward, think about changing your regimen or getting assistance from a healthcare professional.
- Benefits: Changing your workout routine can help avoid hives.

8. Avoid Temperature Extremes

- Instruction: Abrupt temperature changes, such as hot or cold baths or severe weather, can cause hives.

- Benefits: Hives can be avoided by keeping your body temperature steady and pleasant.

9. Stay Hydrated

- Instruction: To stay hydrated, sip lots of water throughout the day.
- Benefits: Staying properly hydrated may lower your chance of developing hives and help you retain healthy skin.

When to Seek Medical Help

- Get help if your hives don't go away, get worse, or show symptoms of an infection (such as increased redness, warmth, or pus).

- Seek emergency medical attention right away if you suffer from severe allergic reactions (anaphylaxis), which include breathing difficulties, facial or neck swelling, or a fast heartbeat.

Methods for Calming and Cooling

Cooling and relaxing methods can relieve itching, swelling, and discomfort, making them useful home treatments for hives (urticaria). These methods can help you properly control your symptoms and calm the affected skin. You can try the following relaxing and cooling methods for hives at home:

1. Cold Compressors

   - Instructions: For ten to fifteen minutes, apply a cold compress—such as an ice pack covered in a thin towel or a cloth soaked in cold water—to the injured area.
   - Benefits: Cold compresses ease discomfort and irritation by numbing the region and reducing swelling.

2. Baths with oatmeal

   - Instructions: Soak for fifteen to twenty minutes in lukewarm bathwater after adding colloidal oatmeal. Using a gentle towel, gently pat dry your skin.
   - Benefits: Because of its calming and anti-inflammatory qualities, oatmeal can help soothe itchy skin.

3. Baking Soda Bath

   - Instructions: Soak for 15 to 20 minutes in a lukewarm bath filled with 1/4 to 1/2 cup baking soda.
   - Benefits: Baking soda can be used to relieve skin irritation and itching.

4. Aloe Vera Gel

   - Instructions: Several times a day, apply pure aloe vera gel directly to the affected region.
   - Benefits: Aloe vera contains anti-inflammatory and cooling qualities that can help soothe irritation and lessen inflammation.

5. Witch Hazel

- Instructions: Use a cotton ball or pad to apply witch hazel extract to the hives.
- Benefits: The astringent and anti-inflammatory qualities of witch hazel can help calm and desiccate hives.

6. Peppermint Tea Compress

- Instructions: Make a cup of peppermint tea, let it cool, then dab a cotton ball or towel over the afflicted area.
- Benefits: Peppermint can help reduce itching and has a cooling impact on the skin.

7. Calamine Lotion

- Instruction: Apply calamine lotion to the hives as needed and allow it to dry on the skin.
- Benefits: Calamine lotion relieves itching and has a cooling effect.

8. Hydration and Moisturization

- Instructions: Use hypoallergenic, fragrance-free moisturizers to keep the skin hydrated and moisturized.
- Benefits: Moisturizing and hydration can help ward off dryness and irritation.

When to Seek Medical Help

- ▷ Get help if your hives don't go away, get worse, or show symptoms of an infection (such as increased redness, warmth, or pus).

- ▷ Seek emergency medical attention right away if you suffer from severe allergic reactions (anaphylaxis), which include breathing difficulties, facial or neck swelling, or an accelerated heartbeat.

Natural Counteragents

Without the need for medicine, natural antihistamines can help manage mild cases of urticaria (hives) by lowering itching and irritation. Use caution when using these natural remedies, especially if you have allergies or sensitivities, even though they might offer relief. Before beginning any new treatment, always get advice from your healthcare professional, particularly if you are taking medication or have a medical condition. Here are some natural antihistamines you can try at home for hives:

1. Quercetin

   - Instructions: One type of flavonoid is quercetin, which can be found in leafy greens, apples, onions, berries, and green tea. You can up your quercetin intake by eating these items.

- Benefits: Because of its anti-inflammatory and antihistamine qualities, quercetin may help lessen hives and allergic reactions.

2. Nettle Tea

- Instructions: Steep dried nettle leaves in boiling water for five to ten minutes to make nettle tea. Throughout the day, sip the tea.
- Benefits: Nettle can help reduce hive symptoms because of its inherent antihistamine qualities.

3. Butterbur

- Instructions: Butterbur is offered as a supplement. For information on the proper dosage, refer to the package instructions or speak with your healthcare provider.
- Benefits: Butterbur can help reduce the symptoms of hives and may contain antihistamine and anti-inflammatory properties.

4. Bromelain

- Instructions: Pineapples contain an enzyme called bromelain. As directed on the packaging, you can either eat fresh pineapple or take a bromelain supplement.
- Benefits: Bromelain can help lessen swelling and irritation and may have anti-inflammatory and antihistamine properties.

5. Vitamin C

- Instructions: Eat more foods high in vitamin C, such as bell peppers, oranges, strawberries, and kiwis, or take a supplement.
- Benefits: Antioxidant vitamin C may strengthen immunity and lessen the intensity of allergic responses.

6. Turmeric

- Instructions: Include turmeric in your meals or take a supplement containing turmeric as directed on the label.
- Benefits: Curcumin, an ingredient in turmeric, has anti-inflammatory and antihistamine qualities that may help lessen the symptoms of hives.

When to Seek Medical Help

- Get help if your hives don't go away, get worse, or show symptoms of an infection (such as increased redness, warmth, or pus).

- Seek emergency medical attention right away if you suffer from severe allergic reactions (anaphylaxis), which include breathing difficulties, facial or neck swelling, or an accelerated heartbeat.

Over-The-Counter Antihistamines and Creams

The itching and pain associated with hives (urticaria) can be relieved with over-the-counter (OTC) antihistamines and treatments. Histamine is a substance that is released during an allergic reaction, and these therapies function by inhibiting its action. When selecting an over-the-counter antihistamine or medication, thoroughly read the label and adhere to the recommended dosage. Here are a few popular over-the-counter antihistamines and hives remedies:

Oral Antihistamines

1. Diphenhydramine (Benadryl)
   - How to Use: Take as directed by the package, usually every four to six hours as needed.
   - Benefits: Diphenhydramine is a potent antihistamine that relieves swelling and itching.

2. Loratadine (Claritin)
   - How to Use: Follow the directions on the package to take one dose each day.
   - Benefits: Loratadine is an antihistamine that doesn't make you sleepy and can help reduce hives symptoms.

3. Cetirizine (Zyrtec)
   - How to Use: Follow the directions on the package to take one dose each day.

- Benefits: Cetirizine effectively relieves hives and itching, while some users may experience slight drowsiness from it.

4. Fexofenadine (Allegra)

- How to Use: Follow the directions on the packaging to take once or twice a day.
- Benefits: Fexofenadine is an antihistamine that doesn't make you sleepy and can help with hives symptoms.

Topical Antihistamines

Diphenhydramine Cream

- How to Use It: As needed, apply a thin coating to the affected region.
- Benefits: Topical diphenhydramine relieves discomfort and irritation in specific areas.

Calamine Lotion

- Use to Use: Apply calamine lotion as needed to the affected region and let it dry on the skin.
- Benefits: Calamine lotion relieves itching and irritation and has a cooling effect.

Hydrocortisone Cream

- How to Use: Up to three times a day, apply a thin coating of 1% hydrocortisone cream to the affected region.
- Benefits: Cream containing hydrocortisone may help lessen itching, redness, and inflammation.

Oatmeal Bath Products

- How to Use: Soak for 15 to 20 minutes in a lukewarm bath using colloidal oatmeal bath products.
- Benefits: Bath products containing oatmeal help calm the skin and reduce inflammation and itching.

When to Seek Medical Help

- Get help if your hives don't go away, get worse, or show symptoms of an infection (such as increased redness, warmth, or pus).

- Seek emergency medical attention right away if you suffer from severe allergic reactions (anaphylaxis), which include breathing difficulties, facial or neck swelling, or an accelerated heartbeat.

CHAPTER 5
LIFESTYLE CHANGES TO MANAGE RASHES AND HIVES

Lifestyle changes can play a significant role in managing skin rashes and hives (urticaria). By making adjustments to your daily routine, you can help prevent flare-ups and reduce symptoms.

Nutrition and Diet

Skin rashes and hives (urticaria) can be effectively managed with dietary and nutritional interventions. Choosing your food carefully can help lessen the frequency and intensity of flare-ups. The following nutritional and dietary approaches can help control rashes and hives:

1. Avoid Known Food Triggers

- Instructions: Recognize and stay away from items, such as nuts, shellfish, eggs, dairy, or specific fruits and vegetables that cause your rashes or hives.
- Benefits: Steering clear of recognized food triggers can help stave off allergic reactions and flare-ups.

2. Maintain a Balanced Diet

- ▷ Instruction: Consume a range of foods high in nutrients, such as whole grains, fruits, vegetables, lean meats, and healthy fats.
- ▷ Benefits: An immune system and general well-being that are supported by a balanced diet can aid in the management of skin disorders.

3. Eat More Foods That Reduce Inflammation

- ▷ Instruction: Include anti-inflammatory foods like leafy greens, almonds, seeds, olive oil, and fatty fish (salmon, mackerel).
- ▷ Benefits: These meals have the potential to alleviate rashes and hives symptoms as well as decrease inflammation.

4. Eat Foods High in Antioxidants

- ▷ Instruction: Incorporate antioxidant-rich foods like dark leafy greens, citrus fruits, berries, and dark chocolate into your diet.
- ▷ Benefits: By defending your skin and immune system, antioxidants may lessen the severity of allergic reactions.

5. Stay Hydrated

- ▷ Instruction: To stay hydrated, sip lots of water throughout the day.

▷ Benefits: Drinking enough water promotes healthy skin and may assist in the treatment of rashes and hives.

6. Monitor Intake of Processed Food

▷ Instruction: Eat less processed and high-sugar foods because these can aggravate inflammation.
▷ Benefits: Cutting back on processed foods can help you feel better overall and manage your symptoms.

7. Probiotics and Prebiotics

▷ Instruction: To improve gut health, include foods high in probiotics (yogurt, kefir, sauerkraut) and prebiotics (onions, garlic, bananas).
▷ Benefits: Your immune system may function better and allergy reactions may be less frequent if your gut is healthy.

8. Consider Vitamin and Minerals Supplements

▷ Instructions: Before taking any supplements, including omega-3 fatty acids, vitamin C, or vitamin D, speak with your doctor.
▷ Benefits: Your immune system may be bolstered and symptoms may be better controlled by certain vitamins and minerals.

When to Seek Medical Help

- If you think that your rashes or hives are being caused by a food allergy, consult a doctor for the appropriate examination and diagnosis.

- See your doctor if, despite dietary adjustments, your symptoms get worse or continue.

Stress Management and Mindfulness

Stress can play a significant role in triggering or exacerbating skin rashes and hives (urticaria). Managing stress and practicing mindfulness can help you maintain overall health and potentially reduce the frequency and severity of flare-ups. Here are some stress management and mindfulness techniques to consider as part of your lifestyle changes to manage rashes and hives:

1. Practice Meditation

- Instruction: Make time daily to meditate, paying attention to your breath and purging all outside distractions from your thoughts.
- Benefits: Stress and tension reduction are two benefits of meditation that may aid with skin issues.

2. Practice Deep Breathing

- ⮞ Instruction: Breathe gently through your nose, hold it for a few seconds, and slowly exhale through your mouth to do deep breathing exercises.
- ⮞ Benefits: You can relieve stress and relax your nervous system by practicing deep breathing.

3. Gradual Relaxation of the Muscles

- ⮞ Instruction: Tense and then release every muscle group in your body, working your way up to your head from your toes.
- ⮞ Benefits: You can induce relaxation and relieve tension by using this technique.

4. Engage in Regular Exercise

- ⮞ Instruction: Include a moderate amount of exercise each day, such as swimming, yoga, or walking.
- ⮞ Benefits: Exercise may assist your skin by lowering stress and enhancing circulation.

5. Get Adequate Sleep.

- ⮞ Instruction: Create a regular sleep routine and try to get between seven and nine hours of sleep every night.

> Benefits: Sleeping well can improve your general health and immune system, which will lessen the negative effects of stress on your skin.

6. Practice Gratitude and Positive Thinking

> Instruction: To keep your attention on the positive aspects of your life, write in a gratitude diary or say positive affirmations every day.
> Benefits: You can feel happier and handle stress better if you think positively.

7. Set Health Boundaries

> Instruction: Recognize when to say no to obligations that may cause you undue stress and put your health first.
> Benefits: You can safeguard your physical and mental well-being and manage stress by establishing healthy limits.

8. Mindful Eating

> Instruction: This technique involves focusing on your meal, eating slowly, and enjoying every bite.
> Benefits: You can become more conscious of your food choices and how they affect your skin by practicing mindful eating.

9. Engage in Relaxing Hobbies

  ⊳ Instructions: Choose enjoyable pastimes for yourself, like gardening, drawing, or reading, and schedule regular time for them.

  ⊳ Benefits: Taking part in enjoyable activities might aid in stress relief and relaxation.

When to Seek Medical Help

- If stress is making it difficult for you to go about your everyday activities or if your symptoms are getting worse, you might want to think about getting help from a professional, like therapy or counseling.

- For additional assessment and treatment, speak with your healthcare physician if your skin problems are worsening or remaining after you have made lifestyle adjustments.

Fabric and Clothes Considerations

Choosing the right clothing and fabrics can help minimize irritation and discomfort for individuals managing rashes and hives (urticaria). Here are some considerations to keep in mind when selecting clothing as part of your lifestyle changes:

1. Choose Clothing That Fits Loosely

  ⊳ Instruction: Opt for loose-fitting attire composed of breathable, soft materials such as linen or cotton.

- ⊳ Benefits: Wearing loose clothing minimizes skin irritation by improving air circulation and reducing friction.

2. Avoid Rough or Irritating Fabrics

- ⊳ Instruction: Avoid wearing materials like wool or harsh synthetics that could irritate delicate skin.
- ⊳ Benefits: Soft, silky textiles are less prone to rub against skin or produce friction.

3. Wear Moisture-Wicking Fabrics for Exercise

- ⊳ Instruction: Choose moisture-wicking clothing, such as blends of polyester, to help wick sweat away from the skin while working out.
- ⊳ Benefits: Fabrics that wick away moisture keep skin dry and lessen the possibility of heat-related rashes or irritation when exercising.

4. Dress in Layers

- ⊳ Instruction: Wear layers of clothing to comfortably transition between different temperatures without being too hot or too cold.
- ⊳ Benefits: Layering reduces the chance of sweating, which can worsen skin irritation, and improves temperature regulation.

5. Choose Hypoallergenic Laundry Detergents

- ▷ Instruction: Wash bedding and clothes with hypoallergenic or fragrance-free laundry detergents.
- ▷ Benefits: These detergents lessen the possibility that textiles contain lingering allergens that could cause skin problems.

6. Wash New Clothes Before Wearing

- ▷ Instruction: Always wash new clothes to get rid of any lingering chemicals or dyes that could irritate skin.
- ▷ Benefits: Cleaning new clothes lowers the possibility of skin reactions by getting rid of possible allergens and irritants.

7. Avoid Wearing Tight or Restrictive Clothing

- ▷ Instruction: Refrain from wearing clothing that is too tight or restrictive since it could produce friction on the skin.
- ▷ Benefits: Loose clothing minimizes the chance of irritation or hives by improving ventilation and lowering pressure on the skin.

8. Take Into Account Wearing Protective Clothing for Outdoor Activities

- ▷ Instruction: Cover up with lightweight, long-sleeved shirts and slacks to protect your skin from the sun and insects.

> Benefits: Wearing protective clothes helps shield the skin from UV rays and insect bites, which can cause allergic reactions in certain people.

When to Seek Medical Help

- See your doctor for additional assessment and treatment if your skin issues are worsening or remaining after you have changed your clothes and way of life.

- Seek emergency medical treatment if you have any of the following symptoms of an allergic reaction: trouble breathing, swelling in the face or throat, or an accelerated heartbeat.

CHAPTER 6

LIVING WELL WITH RASHES AND HIVES

In the chapter, the emphasis is on methods and advice to assist people in controlling their illness and preserving their quality of life even in the face of rashes and hives on the skin (urticaria).

Managing Recurrent or Chronic Symptoms

Although urticaria, or recurrent rashes and hives, can be difficult to manage, there are methods and strategies that people can employ to enhance their quality of life and effectively manage their disease. The following are important details to mention in this section:

1. Acceptance and Mindfulness

- Assist people in learning to accept themselves as they are and to live in the present.

- Encourage the use of mindfulness practices like yoga, deep breathing, and meditation to help control the tension and anxiety brought on by persistent symptoms.

2. Build Coping Skills

- Offer direction on building coping mechanisms to manage the psychological and physical effects of having persistent or recurrent symptoms.

- Provide skills including relaxation methods, positive self-talk, and distraction tactics to assist people in coping with discomfort and keeping an optimistic mindset.

3. Create a Support Network

- Stress the value of asking friends, family, or support groups for assistance as they may provide comprehension, empathy, and motivation.

- Promote open dialogue about treatment alternatives, worries, and any symptom changes with medical professionals.

4. Set Reasonable Expectations

- Assist patients in setting reasonable expectations for the management of their illness, keeping in mind that there could be periods of progress and setbacks.

- Promote adaptation and flexibility in coping mechanisms, acknowledging that what suits one individual may not suit another.

5. Emphasize Self-Care

- Highlight the significance of self-care routines, such as healthy eating, exercise, appropriate skin care, and enough sleep.

- Offer advice on how to prioritize activities that enhance one's physical and mental well-being and incorporate self-care practices into everyday routines.

Seek Professional Support

- Suggest to people that they get help from therapists, counselors, or support groups that focus on dermatological diseases or chronic illnesses.

- Offer information for locating mental health specialists who can help manage the psychological effects of persistent symptoms and provide direction and support.

6. Stay Educated

- Encourage people to learn about triggers, available treatments, and lifestyle changes that can help control symptoms to stay educated about their illness.

- Provide reliable information sources, such as patient advocacy groups, medical websites, and healthcare practitioners.

7. Exercise Self-Compassion

- Motivate people to be kind to themselves and to themselves while they are going through a hard period.

- Remind them that it's acceptable to prioritize taking care of oneself, ask for assistance when needed, and do it without feeling guilty.

Emotional and Mental Health Support

People who suffer from rashes and hives (urticaria) need emotional and mental health care because the condition can negatively affect their quality of life and overall well-being. Here are some essential details to cover under this heading:

1. Psychoeducation

   - Educate people on the psychological and emotional ramifications of having long-term skin problems, particularly how they affect every day functioning, body image, and self-esteem.

   - Provide information and direction on how to comprehend typical emotional responses like stress, anxiety, despair, and impatience.

2. Therapeutic Techniques

   - Provide coping mechanisms and therapeutic approaches to assist people in addressing emotional suffering related to their illness.

- Incorporate methods like journaling, mindfulness-based stress reduction (MBSR), cognitive-behavioral therapy (CBT), and relaxation exercises.

3. Support Groups

- Encourage people to join online communities or support groups for people with long-term skin disorders.

- Give people information on online or local support groups where they can meet people who can relate to their experiences and who can encourage and support them in return.

4. Counseling and Therapy

- Stress the advantages of obtaining expert counseling or therapy to deal with mental and emotional health issues arising from having rashes and hives.

- Provide tools for locating mental health specialists who can offer specialized support and interventions and who have a background in chronic illness or dermatology.

5. Self-Care Practices

- Highlight the significance of self-care activities, such as consistent exercise, a balanced diet, enough sleep, and relaxation methods, for preserving emotional well-being.

- Offer advice on how to prioritize tasks that advance mental and emotional well-being and include self-care activities into everyday routines.

6. Healthful Strategies for Coping

- Encourage people to create healthy coping strategies to deal with stress, worry, and negative emotions. Some of these strategies include being grateful, taking up a hobby, going outside, and looking for social support.

- Provide healthy coping mechanisms as an alternative to substance abuse and avoidance tactics.

7. Self-Acceptance and Compassion

- Stress the value of acceptance and self-compassion in helping people deal with the difficulties of having a chronic skin condition.

- Encourage people to practice self-acceptance and self-love, to be gentle to themselves, and to acknowledge their feelings without passing judgment.

8. Empowerment and Advocacy

- Empower individuals to advocate for themselves in healthcare settings and seek appropriate treatment and support for their emotional and mental health needs.

- Provide resources for staying informed about mental health rights, accessing mental health services, and advocating for better mental health care.

Building a Support Network

Creating a support system is crucial for people with urticaria, or rashes and hives since it offers them social, practical, and emotional assistance to help them manage their illness. The following are important details to mention in this section:

1. Family and Friends

  - Encourage people to ask for help, understanding, and encouragement from their family and friends.

  - Offer advice on how to convey wants and sentiments to loved ones and talk to them about their situation in an effective manner.

2. Online Communities

  - Stress the advantages of joining online groups and discussion boards where people who have gone through similar things can relate to one another, share experiences, and provide support.

  - Offer options for locating trustworthy websites and groups devoted to long-term skin disorders.

3. Support Groups

- Encourage people to join online or locally based support groups for people dealing with chronic skin disorders, rashes, or hives.

- Provide details about local services, activities, and support group gatherings.

4. Patient Advocacy Organizations

- Point people in the direction of nonprofit organizations and patient advocacy organizations that focus on dermatological disorders.

- These groups frequently offer advocacy initiatives, support services, and instructional materials to empower people and increase public awareness of their conditions.

5. Healthcare Providers

- Encourage people to establish a helpful rapport with their medical professionals, such as dermatologists, allergists, and mental health specialists.

- Promote candid dialogue, teamwork, and collaborative decision-making to guarantee that their medical needs are successfully satisfied.

6. Therapeutic Relationships

   - Stress the value of developing therapeutic relationships with medical professionals, therapists, counselors, or support group leaders who have expertise in dermatology or chronic illness.

   - These experts can provide individualized solutions, support, and direction to assist people to manage their conditions and enhance their quality of life.

7. Peer Mentoring Programs

   - Encourage the development of peer mentoring programs in which people who have experienced rashes and hives firsthand can offer others who are just receiving a diagnosis or are having difficulty managing their illness encouragement, direction, and useful information.

   - These initiatives help the community become more resilient, empowered, and supportive of one another.

8. Community Resources

   - Provide details about services and resources in the community, such as wellness initiatives, social gatherings, and educational courses that are accessible to those with long-term skin disorders.

   - Inspire people to look into nearby resources and seize chances to interact with people in their neighborhood.

CONCLUSION

In conclusion, hives and skin rashes are frequent ailments that can be successfully treated with a mix of natural cures and, occasionally, medical attention. People can take proactive measures to manage their skin health and know when to seek professional guidance by being aware of the types, causes, and treatments of skin conditions.